The Complete KETO Drink & Dessert Cooking Guide For Women

Amazing Keto-Friendly Drink & Dessert Recipes To Stay In Shape

Megan Kelly

1

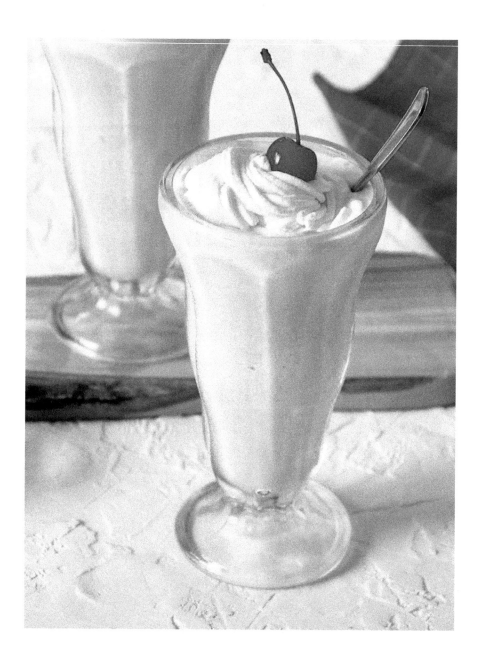

Table of contents

5

Triple Berry Cheesecake Smoothie

Servings: 1

Time: 5 mins

Difficulty: Easy

Nutrients per serving: Calories: 158 kcal | Fat: 11g | Carbohydrates: 12g | Protein: 3g | Fiber: 6g

Ingredients

- 2 Tbsps. Avocado
- 1/2 Cup Mixed Berries, Frozen
- 1 Tsp. Vanilla
- 2 Tbsps. Cream Cheese
- 1/8 Tsp. Sea Salt
- 1/2 Cup Almond Milk, Unsweetened
- 7-10 Drops Monkfruit Extract

Method

1. Combine all the ingredients in a blender and mix until a smooth consistency is attained.
2. Decant into the serving glass and enjoy.

7

Maple Almond Green Smoothie

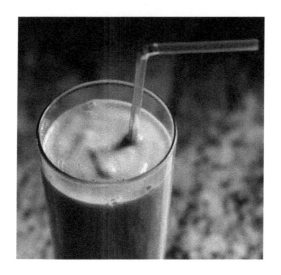

Servings: 1

Time: 5 mins

Difficulty: Easy

Nutrients per serving: Calories: 210 kcal | Fat: 16.8g | Carbohydrates: 10.4g | Protein: 8.1g | Fiber: 6.3g

Ingredients

- 1 Cup Baby Spinach
- 1 Tbsp. Avocado

- 1 Tbsp. Golden Flax Meal
- 1 Tbsp. Almond Butter
- 1 Cup Almond Milk, Unsweetened
- 1 & 1/4 Tsps. Stevia/Erythritol Blend
- 1/4 Tsp. Vanilla Extract
- 1/8 Tsp. Cinnamon
- 1/4 Tsp. Maple Extract
- 2-3 Ice Cubes (Optional)

Method

1. Combine all the ingredients in a blender and mix until a smooth consistency is attained.
2. Decant into the serving glass and enjoy.

Dairy Free Chocolate Pecan Keto Shake

Servings: 1

Time: 10 mins

Difficulty: Easy

Nutrients per serving: Calories: 247 kcal | Fat: 20g | Carbohydrates: 12g | Protein: 5g | Fiber: 8g

Ingredients

- 5 Raw Pecans, Halved
- 2 Tbsps. Cocoa Powder, Unsweetened
- 1/8 Tsp. Pink Himalayan Salt
- 1 & 1/3 Cups Almond Milk, Unsweetened
- 2 & 1/2 Tsps. Stevia/Erythritol Blend
- 2 Tbsps. Avocado
- 3-4 Ice Cubes

Method

1. Combine all the ingredients in a blender and mix until a smooth consistency is attained.
2. Decant into the serving glass and enjoy.

Strawberry Colada Milkshake

Servings: 1

Time: 3 mins

Difficulty: Easy

Nutrients per serving: Calories: 660 kcal | Fat: 60g | Carbohydrates: 7g | Protein: 13g | Fiber: 7g

Ingredients

- 1/2 Tbsp. Chia Seeds
- 3-4 Strawberries, Frozen
- 1/3 Cup Coconut Milk
- 1/3 Cup Almond Milk, Unsweetened
- 1 Tsp. Stevia/Erythritol Blend
- 4-5 Ice Cubes
- 1/8 Tsp. Pink Salt
- 1/4 Tsp. Coconut Extract
- 1/4 Tsp. Vanilla Extract
- 1/2 Tbsp. Coconut Oil (Optional)
- 1 Tbsp. Strawberries, Freeze-Dried (Optional)

Method

1. Combine all the ingredients in a blender and mix until a smooth consistency is attained.
2. Decant into the serving glass and enjoy.

Keto Frozen Hot Chocolate

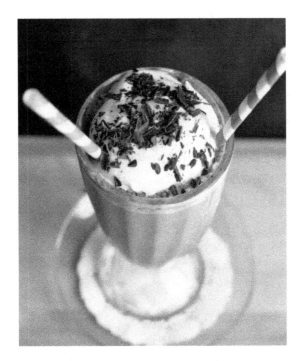

Servings: 1

Time: 5 mins

Difficulty: Easy

Nutrients per serving: Calories: 660 kcal | Fat: 60g | Carbohydrates: 7g | Protein: 13g | Fiber: 7g

Ingredients

- 1 Tbsp. Avocado
- 1/4 Cup Coconut Milk
- 1 Tbsp. Cocoa
- 1/2 Cup Almond Milk, Unsweetened
- 1/2 Cup Ice Cubes
- 1 & 1/4 Tsps. Stevia/Erythritol Blend
- 1/2 Tsp. Vanilla
- 1/8 Tsp. Pink Himalayan Salt

For Garnish

- Chocolate Chips, Sugar-Free
- Whipped Coconut Cream

Method

1. Combine all the ingredients in a blender except ice cubes. Blend until a smooth consistency is attained.
2. Decant into the serving glass, add the ice, and put the whipped cream and chocolate chips on top if you want.

Dairy-Free Keto Iced Latte

Servings: 1

Time: 5 mins

Difficulty: Easy

Nutrients per serving: Calories: 660 kcal | Fat: 60g | Carbohydrates: 7g | Protein: 13g | Fiber: 7g

Ingredients

- 1/4 Cup Brewed Coffee, Strong
- 1 & 1/2 Cups Almond Milk, Unsweetened
- 1 Tbsp. MCT Oil

Method

1. Brew your coffee according to your preference.
2. Combine all the ingredients in a blender and mix until a smooth consistency is attained.
3. Decant into the serving cup and enjoy.

Sugar-Free Hibiscus Lemonade

Servings: 4

Time: 10 mins

Difficulty: Easy

Nutrients per serving: Calories: 660 kcal | Fat: 60g | Carbohydrates: 7g | Protein: 13g | Fiber: 7g

Ingredients

- 1 & 1/2 Cups Sparkling Mineral Water
- 2 Tbsps. Lemon Juice, Fresh
- 1 Tbsp. Stevia/Erythritol Blend
- 2 Cups Brewed Hibiscus Tea
- Ice, To Taste

Method

1. Put all the ingredients in a pitcher except water and ice. Mix everything well until dissolved.
2. Add the water and ice and stir.
3. Decant into the serving glasses and enjoy.

Low Carb 7Up

Servings: 2

Time: 2 mins

Difficulty: Easy

Nutrients per serving: Calories: 2 kcal | Fat: 0g | Carbohydrates: 1g | Protein: 0g | Fiber: 0g

Ingredients

- 1 & 1/2 Cups Ice
- 1/4 Tsp. Liquid Stevia
- 1/2 Tbsp. Lime Juice
- 2/3 Cup Seltzer Water

Method

1. Fill serving glass with ice and put all the other ingredients in it.
2. Stir well and enjoy.

Low Carb German Chocolate Fat Bomb Hot Chocolate

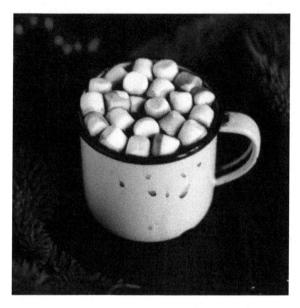

Servings: 1

Time: 12 mins

Difficulty: Easy

Nutrients per serving: Calories: 358 kcal | Fat: 39g | Carbohydrates: 2g | Protein: 2g

Ingredients

- 2 Tbsps. Cocoa Butter
- 1/4 Cup Coconut Milk
- 1 Cup Chocolate Almond Milk, Unsweetened
- Stevia, To Taste

Method

1. In a saucepan, combine all the ingredients and heat over medium-low flame until the cocoa butter melts.
2. Remove from the heat and mix with an immersion blender till t becomes frothy.
3. Decant into your favorite mug and enjoy.

Low Carb German Gingerbread Hot Chocolate

Servings: 2

Time: 20 mins

Difficulty: Easy

Nutrients per serving: Calories: 72 kcal | Fat: 4g | Carbohydrates: 11g | Protein: 3g | Fiber: 5g

Ingredients

- 1/4 Cup Cocoa Powder, Unsweetened
- 2 Cups Chocolate Almond Milk, Unsweetened
- 1/2 Tsp. Liquid Stevia
- 1/4 Cup Stevia
- 1/4 Tsp. Cardamom, Ground
- 1 Tsp. Cinnamon, Ground
- 1/8 Tsp. Allspice, Ground
- 1/8 Tsp. Anise Seed, Ground
- 1/8 Tsp. Cloves, Ground
- 1/8 Tsp. Nutmeg, Ground
- 1/8 Tsp. Ginger, Ground

Method

1. Combine all the ingredients in a saucepan and heat it over medium heat.
2. Once it boils, reduce the heat to low, and let it simmer for about 5 minutes with intermittent stirring.
3. Decant into serving mugs and enjoy.

Coconut Pumpkin Steamer

Servings: 1

Time: 5 mins

Difficulty: Easy

Nutrients per serving: Calories: 241 kcal | Fat: 24g | Carbohydrates: 9g | Protein: 2g | Fiber: 1g

Ingredients

- 1 Tsp. Vanilla Extract
- 1/2 Cup Coconut Milk
- Stevia, To Taste
- 1/4 Tsp. Pumpkin Pie Spice, Without Sugar

Method

1. Combine all the ingredients in a saucepan and heat it over medium heat.
2. Once the bubbles start to form, take off the heat, and serve warm.

Low Carb Margarita Mix

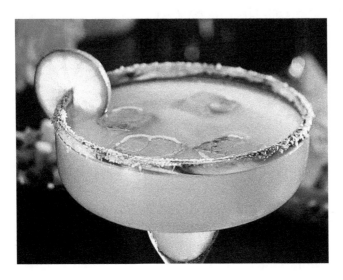

Servings: 2

Time: 5 mins

Difficulty: Easy

Nutrients per serving: Calories: 35 kcal | Fat: 0g | Carbohydrates: 9g | Protein: 0g | Fiber: 0g

Ingredients

- 1/2 Cup Lemon Juice, Fresh
- 1 & 1/2 Cups Water

- 1/4 Tsp. Liquid Stevia
- 1/3 Cup Erythritol, Powdered
- 1/8 Tsp. Orange Extract
- 1 Cup Tequila
- Ice, To Taste

Method

1. Combine all the ingredients in a pitcher except tequila and ice.
2. Mix well to dissolve the sweetener.
3. Add the tequila and stir.
4. Pour in the cocktail glasses with rims covered with salt.
5. Add the ice and enjoy.

Low Carb Electrolyte Water

Servings: 4

Time: 5 mins

Difficulty: Easy

Nutrients per serving: Calories: 2 kcal | Fat: 0g | Carbohydrates: 1g | Protein: 0g

Ingredients

- 4 Cups Water
- 2 Tbsps. Lemon Juice
- 1/8 Tsp. Baking Soda
- Stevia, To Taste
- 1/8 Tsp. Salt

Method

1. Combine all the ingredients in a bottle, cover it, and shake well.
2. Serve and enjoy.

Low Carb Pumpkin Spice Mocha

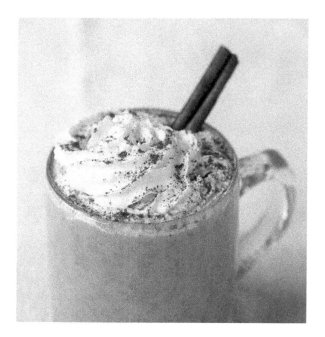

Servings: 2

Time: 15 mins

Difficulty: Easy

Nutrients per serving: Calories: 187 kcal | Fat: 21g | Carbohydrates: 1g | Protein: 0g

Ingredients

- 1 Tsp. Pumpkin Pie Spice, Without Sugar
- Stevia, To Taste
- 3 Tbsps. Cocoa Butter
- 1/4 Cup Coffee Grounds
- 3 Cups Water

Method

1. Brew the coffee according to your preference with the pumpkin spice in it.
2. Add the cocoa butter in it and blend with an immersion blender until a smooth consistency is attained and it becomes frothy.
3. Add the desired quantity of sweetener and enjoy.

Kombucha Sangria

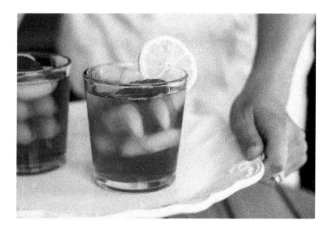

Servings: 7

Time: 10 mins

Difficulty: Easy

Nutrients per serving: Calories: 101 kcal | Fat: 0g | Carbohydrates: 6.5g | Protein: 0.1g | Fiber: 0g

Ingredients

- 4 Tbsps. Monkfruit, Powdered
- 1 Cup Orange Juice
- 2 Cups Kombucha
- 3 & 1/4 Cups Spanish Wine

- 1 Lime, Sliced
- 1 Orange, Sliced
- 1 Lemon, Sliced
- 1/2 Cup Brandy (Optional)

Method

1. Combine all the ingredients in a pitcher, except orange, lemon, and lime slices.
2. Stir well to mix and add the orange, lemon, and lime slices.
3. Serve with ice and enjoy.

Pumpkin Spice Hot Buttered Rum

Servings: 4

Time: 10 mins

Difficulty: Easy

Nutrients per serving: Calories: 73 kcal | Fat: 60g | Carbohydrates: 1.2g | Protein: 0.2g | Fiber: 0.5g

Ingredients

- 1 Cup Butter
- 1 Cup Golden Monkfruit
- 3 Tbsps. Maple Syrup, Sugar-Free
- 2 Tsps. Vanilla Extract
- 1 Cup Heavy Cream
- 1 & 1/2 Cups Monkfruit, Powdered
- 1 Tbsp. Pumpkin Pie Spice
- 2 Cups Hot Water
- 1 Cup Rum

Method

1. Take a bowl and put the golden Monkfruit, butter, vanilla, and maple syrup in it. Whisk well for few minutes until creamy and fluffy.
2. Add all the other ingredients except rum and water and mix well. Set aside.
3. Fill each serving glass with 1/4 cup Rum, 1/2 cup water, and two to three tbsps. of the batter and stir well.

Tart Cherry Lemon Drop

Servings: 1

Time: 5 mins

Difficulty: Easy

Nutrients per serving: Calories: 660 kcal | Fat: 60g | Carbohydrates: 7g | Protein: 13g | Fiber: 7g

Ingredients

- 4 Tbsps. Tart Cherry Juice
- 4 Lemon Wedges
- 2 Tbsps. Fresh Lemon Juice
- 3 Tbsps. Vodka
- 2 Tbsps. Water
- 1 Tbsp. Monkfruit, Powdered
- 1 Tbsp. Lemon Juice, Fresh
- 1 Tsp. Monkfruit, Granular
- Ice, To Taste

Method

1. Combine powdered lemon juice, water, and lemon wedges in a blender and blend well until a smooth consistency is attained.
2. Add the vodka, tart cherry juice, and ice in it and blend again until desires consistency.
3. Dip the rim of the cocktail glass in lemon juice and then in granular Monkfruit.
4. Pour in the juice and garnish with a lemon slice if you want.

Orange Creamsicle Mimosas

Servings: 1

Time: 10 mins

Difficulty: Easy

Nutrients per serving: Calories: 255 kcal | Fat: 11.5g | Carbohydrates: 8g | Protein: 0.9g | Fiber: 0.1g

Ingredients

- 1 Tbsp. Vanilla Vodka
- 1/4 Cup Orange Juice, Fresh
- 2 Tbsps. Heavy Cream
- 1 Tsp. Monkfruit, Powdered
- 1/2 Cup Sparkling Wine, Dry (Prosecco Or Champagne)

Method

1. Combine all the ingredients in a blender except wine. Blend it well until a smooth consistency is attained.
2. Add the wine and serve.

Low Carb Strawberry Basil Bourbon Smash

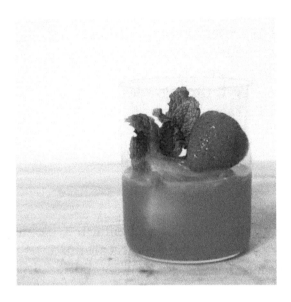

Servings: 1

Time: 10 mins

Difficulty: Easy

Nutrients per serving: Calories: 159 kcal | Fat: 0.4g | Carbohydrates: 3.5g | Protein: 0.5g | Fiber: 0.9g

Ingredients

- 1/4 Cup Bourbon
- 3 Basil Leaves
- 1/8 Tsp. Black Pepper, Ground
- 3 Strawberries, Sliced
- 2 Tbsps. Lemon Juice, Fresh
- 1 Tsp. Erythritol, Powdered
- Ice, To Taste

Method

1. Combine all the ingredients in a blender and blend until desired consistency is attained.
2. Decant in serving glass and enjoy.

Sugar-Free Keto Blueberry Muffins With Almond Flour

Servings: 12

Time: 45 mins

Difficulty: Easy

Nutrients per serving: Calories: 247 kcal | Fat: 21.8g | Carbohydrates: 9.3g | Protein: 7.3g | Fiber: 3.9g

Ingredients

- 1 Tbsp of Baking powder
- 1 tsp of Sea salt
- 1/2 Cup Unsweetened Applesauce
- 2 tsp Vanilla extract
- 2/3 Cup Fresh blueberries
- 3 Cups Almond flour
- 1 tsp Baking soda
- 3 Large Eggs, at room temperature
- 3/4 cup of Monkfruit (or granulated sweetener of choice)
- 4 Tbsp Coconut flour, packed
- 7 Tbsp Coconut oil, melted

Method

1. Preheat the oven to 350 F and use an oil spray to spray a muffin pan.
2. Mix the coconut flour, almond flour, baking powder, baking soda, and salt in a medium dish. Just put aside.
3. In a wide cup, beat together the coconut oil, eggs, monk fruit, applesauce, and vanilla until well mixed, using the electric hand mixer.
4. Stir in the mixture of almond flour until well mixed, together with the blueberries. Let a batter stand for 5 minutes so the moisture can continue to be absorbed by the coconut flour.
5. Divide into 12 muffin cavities (use a large ice cream scoop for cooking the muffins with very domed tops) and bake until clean, approximately 24-25 minutes, golden brown, and insert a toothpick in the middle comes out.
6. Leave for 15 minutes to cool. Then, to remove them, loop a knife carefully along the sides of each muffin. Then, before attempting to take them out, let them cool perfectly in the pan.

Keto Zucchini Muffins With Almond Flour

Servings: 12

Time: 30 mins

Difficulty: Easy

Nutrients per serving: Calories: 217 kcal | Fat: 18.5g | Carbohydrates: 8.6g | Protein: 8.2g | Fiber: 4g

Ingredients

- 1 1/2 Cups Monk fruit sweetener
- 1 Tbsp Ground Cardamom
- 1 Tbsp Ground cinnamon
- 1 tsp Baking soda
- 1 tsp Salt
- 1 tsp Vanilla extract
- 1/2 cup Tahini
- 2 Cups Grated zucchini, packed (about 2 medium zucchinis)
- 2 Large Eggs
- 2 tsp Baking powder
- 3 Cups Almond meal (10.5 oz)
- 5 Tbsp Unsweetened vanilla almond milk

Method

1. Preheat the oven to 350 F and adjust to one position below the oven rack center. Use cooking spray to spray a muffin pan.
2. Stir the almond meal, cardamom, baking powder, cinnamon, salt, and soda together in a medium bowl and set aside.
3. Using the electric hand mixer, mix the monk fruit, tahini, almond milk, eggs, and vanilla extract in a large bowl until well mixed.
4. The wet mixture adds the dry mixture and stirs until well mixed, and a thick batter emerges. Finally, fold in a grated zucchini softly when mixed uniformly.
5. Divide the mixture, filling up to the tip, into 12 muffin cavities. I like to use a huge scoop of ice cream, as it gives them a very good, domed top.
6. Bake for about 20-22 minutes, until a toothpick put in the middle, comes out clean. Let it cool for 10 minutes in the bath. Next, turn to a wire rack to cool off perfectly.

Sugar-Free Low Carb Keto Pecan Pie

Servings: 12

Time: 1 day 55 mins

Difficulty: Easy

Nutrients per serving: Calories: 328.7 kcal | Fat: 31.1g | Carbohydrates: 18.8g | Protein: 5g | Fiber: 2.7g

Ingredients

- 6 Tbsp Unsalted butter
- 3/4 tsp Salt
- 2/3 cup Powdered erythritol sweetener (I used swerve)
- 2 large eggs
- 1 tsp Vanilla
- 1 tsp Maple extract
- 1 Almond flour pie crust
- 1 1/4 Cups Heavy whipping cream
- 1 1/2 Cups Pecans

Method

1. Whisk together all the sweetener and the butter in a big, high-sided frying pan set over medium-low heat. Cook, constantly whisking, until golden brown in the mixture, around 5-7 minutes.
2. When whisking continuously, throw in the creamy until golden and carry to a soft simmer.
3. Simmer, constantly stirring, around 8 minutes, until the mixture only starts to thicken. Remove from the heat and allow 30 minutes to cool.
4. Heat your oven to 350 F as it is cooling, then spread the pecans on the large baking sheet. Bake until browned and toasted for 10-12 minutes. Then, cut them loose and set them aside.
5. Add in eggs, salt, and the extracts and stir until smooth, until the mixture is cooled somewhat. Stir the pecans in.
6. Through the cooled pie crust, pour the filling and bake until the top feels firm, about 30 minutes. Let it cool at room temperature and cover overnight, and refrigerate.
7. Slice and devour the next day.

Low Carb Keto Mug Cake

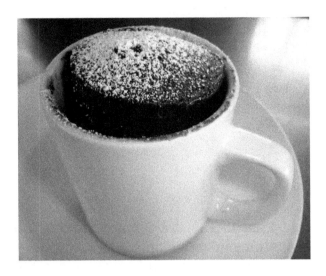

Servings: 1

Time: 8 mins

Difficulty: Easy

Nutrients per serving: Calories: 312 kcal | Fat: 23.9g | Carbohydrates: 19.6g | Protein: 8.2g | Fiber: 11.6g

Ingredients

- 1 Egg yolk
- 1 Tbsp Coconut oil, melted

- 1 tsp Sugar-free chocolate chips
- 1/2 tsp Baking powder
- 1/2 tsp Vanilla extract
- 2 1/2 Tbsp Monkfruit sweetener
- 2 Tbsp Unsweetened cocoa powder
- 3 Tbsp Coconut flour
- 5 Tbsp Unsweetened vanilla almond milk
- Pinch of salt

Method

1. Whisk all of the dried ingredients in a small dish (everything up to the milk.)
2. Stir the remaining ingredients, minus the chocolate chips, in a separate, shallow cup. Pour in the dry ingredients and stir until the mixture is tender. Stir the chips in.
3. Transfer to a wide mug (14-16oz at least) and distributed evenly.
4. Cook it until the top is fixed and it is no bigger than a dime on some wet spots.

Keto Chocolate Peanut Butter Fat Bombs

Servings: 12

Time: 1 hr 10 mins

Difficulty: Easy

Nutrients per serving: Calories: 127 kcal | Fat: 11.6g | Carbohydrates: 3.7g | Protein: 3.8g | Fiber: 1.4g

Ingredients

- 30-40 Drops Liquid stevia (to taste)
- 3/4 Cup Natural creamy peanut butter (may also use almond butter)
- 3 Tbsp cocoa powder (Unsweetened)
- 3 Tbsp Coconut oil

Method

1. Line a mini muffin tin with liners for mini muffins.
2. In a big, microwave-safe dish, put the coconut oil and peanut butter and heat until smooth and molten, for about 1 min.

3. Whisk in the powder with the chocolate until smooth. Then, to taste, whisk the stevia in.
4. Cover about 3/4 of the way, complete with the muffin cavities. Place the pan gently in the refrigerator and cool for around 1 hour, until solid.

Black Walnut Chocolate Chip Muffins With Almond Flour

Servings: 12

Time: 40 mins

Difficulty: Easy

Nutrients per serving: Calories: 292 kcal | Fat: 26.1g | Carbohydrates: 10.9g | Protein: 8.3g | Fiber: 5.8g

Ingredients

- 1 Tbsp of Baking powder
- 1 Tbsp Vanilla extract
- 1 tsp of Baking soda
- 1/2 cup + 1 Tbsp Stevia-sweetened chocolate chips
- 1/4 Cup Hammons Black Walnuts, diced
- 3 cups Almond flour (300g)
- 3 large eggs, at room temperature (important)
- 3/4 cup of Monkfruit
- 1 tsp of Salt
- 4 Tbsp Coconut flour, firmly packed (32g)
- 6 Tbsp of Full-fat coconut milk (canned)
- 6 Tbsp of melted Ghee

Method

1. Preheat the oven to 350 °F and coat a muffin pan generously with cooking spray.
2. Mix the almond flour, baking powder, coconut flour, baking soda, and salt in a big dish.
3. Beat the monk fruit, coconut milk, eggs, ghee, and vanilla in a wide cup, using the electric hand mixer, until well mixed.
4. Add the mixture of flour and whisk until it is well mixed. Stir in the black walnuts and chocolate chips. It's going to be moist for your combination, much like cookie dough. Then sit for 5 mins so that the moisture can start to absorb the coconut flour.
5. Fill your muffin tin around 2/3 of the way (we like to use ice cream scoop to make the muffins look cool and domed) and bake on until tops are golden brown, about 25-27 minutes, and insert a toothpick in the middle comes out clean.
6. Let the cool pan Full. Then, loosen them with a knife along each muffin's edges and separate them from the tray.

Keto Pumpkin Cheesecake

Servings: 12

Time: 2 hrs 20 mins

Difficulty: Easy

Nutrients per serving: Calories: 242 kcal | Fat: 23g | Carbohydrates: 5.7g | Protein: 6.5g | Fiber: 1.5g

Ingredients

- 3/4 cup Monkfruit
- 2/3 Cup Canned pumpkin
- 2 large eggs, at room temp
- 16 Oz Full fat cream cheese, at room temperature (2 blocks)
- 1 Tbsp Vanilla extract
- 1 Tbsp Pumpkin Pie Spice
- 1 Gluten-free Graham Cracker Crust, baked in a 9-inch springform pan

Method

1. Preheat up to 325 °F in your oven.

2. Beat the cream cheese and the monk fruit together in a large bowl using the electric hand mixer until smooth and well mixed.
3. Include all the ingredients, then beat until they are mixed. Don't beat it too hard, or the entrance of too much air in the cheesecake will cause it to sink during baking.
4. With 2 or 3 layers of tinfoil, take the graham cracker crust first from the freezer and then wrap the bottom and the sides very firmly. Place the pan in a large pan for roasting.
5. Onto the crust, pour the cheesecake, and smooth out uniformly. Switch to your oven's middle rack and cover the pan with water until the springform pan comes halfway up.
6. Bake for about 55-60 minutes, until the outside is set and a little circle in the middle is jiggly. Turn the oven off and gently break the lock, allowing the cheesecake to sit for 15 minutes in the oven. Shift to the counter to cool fully, then.
7. Cover up and refrigerate for 8 hours until cool, but better if overnight.
8. Hover a knife down the sides of a cheesecake softly, cut the pan and slice it out.

Sugar-Free No-Bake Keto Cheesecake

Servings: 2

Time: 5 mins

Difficulty: Easy

Nutrients per serving: Calories: 292 kcal | Fat: 28g | Carbohydrates: 4.9g | Protein: 8g | Fiber: 0.9g

Ingredients

For The Crust:

- 1 tsp Powdered Erythritol Sweetener (I used Swerve)
- 2 tsp Ghee or butter, melted
- 3 Tbsp Almond flour, packed

The Cheesecake:

- 0.5 Cup Cream cheese (softened to room temperature)
- 0.5 tsp Vanilla extract
- 8-12 tsp of Powdered Erythritol Sweetener (to taste)
- 4 Tbsp 2% Plain Greek yogurt

Method

1. Stir the almond flour with sweetener together in a shallow dish. In the ghee, add in and mix until crumbly. Push a tiny ramekin onto the rim.
2. Beat a cream cheese plus sweetener in a medium bowl using the electric hand mixer. Add Cream cheese and vanilla, then beat until mixed again, keeping the sides from scraping as desired.
3. To taste sugar again. Spoon over crust and smoothly spread out. To firm up cream cheese, cool for at least 2 hours.

Sugar-Free Keto Lemon Bars

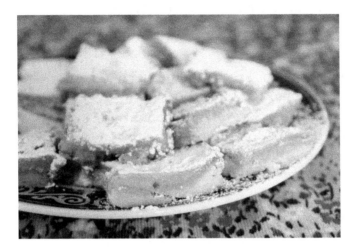

Servings: 16

Time: 1 hr 25 mins

Difficulty: Easy

Nutrients per serving: Calories: 106 kcal | Fat: 8.9g | Carbohydrates: 4.7g | Protein: 2.5g | Fiber: 2.3g

Ingredients

For The Crust:

- Pinch of salt

- 2 Tbsp Monkfruit
- 1/2 cup Coconut oil
- 1 cup of Coconut flour (95g)

For The Topping:

- 3/4 Cup Fresh lemon juice (about 6 large juicy lemons)
- 1 1/2 tsp Coconut flour, sifted
- 1/2 cup Monkfruit
- 2 tsp of Lemon zest
- 4 Eggs

Method

1. Preheat oven to 350 °F and use coconut oil to generously oil an 8x8 inch pan. Only put aside.
2. Include the coconut flour until it forms a dough.
3. Press the dough uniformly into the pan and bake for about 10 minutes, until just slightly golden brown.
4. Carefully stir together the lemon zest and eggs in a wide bowl until the crust has cooled.

Keto Brownies

Servings: 16

Time: 30 mins

Difficulty: Easy

Nutrients per serving: Calories: 107 kcal | Fat: 10g | Carbohydrates: 5.7g | Protein: 2.5g | Fiber: 2.9g

Ingredients

- 1 large egg
- 1/2 tsp Baking soda
- 1/2 tsp Mint extract
- 1/4 cup Plant-based chocolate protein powder
- 1/4 tsp Sea salt
- 2 Egg yolks
- 2 Tbsp vanilla almond milk (Unsweetened)
- 5 ounces Sugar-free chocolate (roughly chopped and divided)
- 6 Tbsp Erythritol Sweetener
- 7 Tbsp Coconut oil (melted and divided)

Method

1. Preheat the oven to 350 °F and use coconut oil to generously oil an 8x8 inch pan. Put aside.
2. Beat the coconut oil and monk fruit and a pinch of salt together in a large bowl, using an electric hand mixer, until smooth and well mixed. Include coconut flour until it forms a dough.
3. Press the dough uniformly into the pan and bake for about 10 minutes, until just softly golden brown. Leave to cool for 30 minutes.
4. Lower the oven temperature to 325 °F and make sure that the oven rack is in the center of the oven.
5. Carefully stir together the lemon zest and eggs in a wide bowl until the crust has cooled. Don't use an electric blender here, or once fried, you can top with crack.
6. Heat the lemon juice softly in a separate, medium dish. Whisk in and stir in the monk fruit until it is dissolved. At room temperature, let it cool fully.

Peanut Butter Truffles

Servings: 10 Truffles

Time: 30 mins

Difficulty: Easy

Nutrients per serving (2 Truffles): Calories: 132 kcal | Fat: 9.9g | Carbohydrates: 10.9g | Protein: 4.4g | Fiber: 5.6g

Ingredients

- 2 tbsp Choc Zero Vanilla Syrup (Sugar-Free)
- 1/4 cup peanut butter
- 1/4 cup Coconut flour
- 1/3 cup chocolate chips (sugar-free)

Method

1. Mix all the peanut butter and the sugar-free syrup in a medium-sized dish.
2. To mix, add the coconut flour and mix. You are looking for a quality that you can roll into balls quickly. You can change the consistency if it is too moist or too dry

by adding more coconut flour or the sweetener if required.

3. Take heaped Tsp. fuls of the blend and roll between your hands into balls. Move them to a plate or tray lined with paper that is oil proof.
4. Place the truffles for 10-20 minutes in the freezer until they are solid.
5. Melt the chocolate chips, meanwhile.
6. Take the truffles from the fridge and use the chocolate to decorate them. You should dip them in full or drizzle on top with a little chocolate-up it's to you.
7. For up to 1 week, you can store it in the refrigerator.

Creamy Keto Chia Pudding

Servings: 2

Time: 6 hrs 10 mins

Difficulty: Easy

Nutrients per serving: Calories: 258 kcal | Fat: 18g | Carbohydrates: 8.15g | Protein: 3.66g | Fiber: 4.3g

Ingredients

- 1 cup Coconut milk full-fat
- 1 dash Salt
- 1/4 tsp Vanilla extract
- 1/4-1/2 tsp Stevia glycerite
- 2 tbsp Sugar-free jam
- 3 tbsp Black chia seeds

Method

1. In a small mug, mix the chia seeds and 1/2 cup of coconut milk.

2. Whisk together the vanilla, salt, and the leftover coconut milk. Use your preferred liquid sweetener to sweeten the flavor.
3. After 30 minutes, refrigerate and stir well to avoid Chia seeds from clumping at the bottom of the container. Overnight, refrigerate.
4. Layer the chia pudding in a serving cup or a small compact container of 1 Tbsp. of sugar-free jelly. Store in your refrigerator for up to 5 days.

Cranberry Almond Crumb Muffins

Servings: 12

Time: 40 mins

Difficulty: Easy

Nutrients per serving: Calories: 330 kcal | Fat: 28.73g | Carbohydrates: 9.46g | Protein: 8.12g | Fiber: 5g

Ingredients

Dry Ingredients (divided use)

- 1/2 cup coconut flour (50 g)
- 1/2 cup low carb sugar (115 g)
- 1/2 Tsp. baking soda
- 1/2 Tsp. salt
- 1 1/2 cups fresh cranberries chopped, (115 g)
- 2 cups almond flour (185 g)
- 2 Tsp. baking powder
- 2 Tbsp. psyllium husk powder (20 gm)

Wet Ingredients

- 6 large eggs
- 1 Tsp. vanilla extract
- 1 Tbsp. white vinegar

- 1/2 Tsp. stevia glycerite
- 1/2 Tsp. almond extract
- 1/2 cup full-fat coconut milk (118 ml)

<u>Crumb Mixture</u>

- 1/4 cup sliced almonds a small handful
- 1/3 cup reserved dry ingredients (35 g)
- 2 Tbsp. low carb sugar
- 1 Tbsp. coconut oil melted (or butter)

Method

1. Preheat the oven to 350 °F and raise the lower third of the rack.
2. With the paper liners, line a muffin pan or brush well with the baking spray. °F
3. Dry Ingredients: Weigh into a medium bowl the first 6 ingredients - NOT the psyllium husk powder.
4. To break up any lumps and to spread the ingredients equally, whisk well.
5. Drop 1/3 cup of the dry mixture and place it in a small dish.
6. To add the muffin ingredients, add the psyllium husk powder and stir again.
7. On top, pour the chopped cranberries.
8. If the tops are well browned, insert a toothpick into the center of a muffin comes out clean, and the cranberry muffins are finished.

Buttery Keto Pecan Sandies Cookies

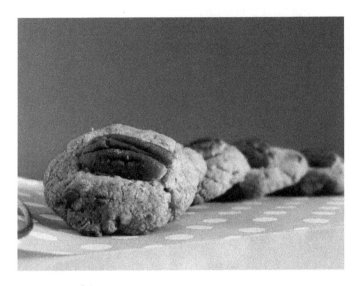

Servings: 18 cookies

Time: 1 hr 22 mins

Difficulty: Easy

Nutrients per serving: Calories: 126 kcal | Fat: 12.16g | Carbohydrates: 3.2g | Protein: 2.33g | Fiber: 2.4g

Ingredients

- 1 1/2 tsp Xanthan gum

- 1 cup Almond flour (90 g)
- 1 cup Pecans (4 oz/ 113 g)
- 1 Egg white beaten
- 1 tsp Vanilla
- 1/2 cup Low carb sugar (90 g)
- 1/2 cup Oat fiber (34 g)
- 1/4 tsp Baking soda
- 2 tsp Gelatin (optional)
- 8 tbsp cold salted butter cut into small pieces
- Extra sweetener for dipping tops (2 tbsp)

Method

1. Preheat the oven to 350 and place the rack in the center position. Using parchment paper to cover a sheet pan.
2. Pour pecans and cut them into tiny pieces in the food processor.
3. To combine, add the next Six ingredients and mix.
4. Cut butter into the small pieces and add it until put into the food processor, grinding.
5. Beat vanilla into the white egg in a tiny cup.
6. The food processor spread the mixture equally all around ingredients and pulse until the dough is uniformly moist.

Keto Cranberry Crumb Bars

Servings: 16

Time: 1 hr

Difficulty: Easy

Nutrients per serving: Calories: 196 kcal | Fat: 14g | Carbohydrates: 8g| Protein: 4g | Fiber: 3g

Ingredients

Cranberry Filling
- 1 cup water (236.58 g)
- 1 pinch fresh ground nutmeg
- 1 pinch salt
- 1 Tbsp. lemon juice (15 ml) or 3 Real Lemon packets
- 1/2 cup low carbohydrates powdered sugar (80 g)
- 12 ounces cranberries (340 g) fresh or frozen

Shortbread Crust
- 2 cups almond flour (180 g)
- 1 cup shredded coconut (90 g) ground in a coffee grinder
- 1/3 cup whey protein powder (20 g)
- 1/3 cup low carb powdered sugar (50 g)

- 1/2 Tsp. salt
- 8 Tbsp. salted butter melted

Crumb Topping

- 3/4 cup of a shortbread crust mixture
- 1/2 cup chopped walnuts (40 g)
- 3 Tbsp. Low carb brown sugar (35 g)
- 3 Tbsp. Sugar-Free Chocolate Chips (40 g)

Method

1. By cutting a parchment's strips large enough to fill the pan's bottom and go up to two respective ends and hangover, prepare an 8x8 or 9x9 brownie pan.
2. With baking spray, spray the pan and placed the piece of parchment in the pan, smoothing it to match. Then you have to chop the walnuts.
3. Place all of the cranberry filling ingredients in a medium pot and bring it to a boil.
4. For 10-15 minutes, simmer gently until a mixture thickens.
5. When the cranberries are frying, process the crushed coconut until it is finely ground in a coffee grinder or small food processor.
6. In a medium dish, place all the dry ingredients for a shortbread crust.
7. The butter is warmed and poured over the dry ingredients.

Low Carb Apple Crumb Muffins

Servings: 12

Time: 45 mins

Difficulty: Easy

Nutrients per serving: Calories: 155 kcal | Fat: 12g | Carbohydrates: 9g | Protein: 5.86g | Fiber: 5.6g

Ingredients

Dry Ingredients (divided use)

- 2 cups Almond flour (190 g)
- 2 tsp Baking powder
- 1/2 cup Oat fiber (45 g)
- 1/2 cup Low Carb Brown Sugar (80 g)
- 1/2 tsp Baking soda
- 1/2 tsp Xanthan gum
- 1/2 tsp ground cardamom
- 1/4 tsp Allspice
- 1/4 tsp ground ginger
- 1/4 tsp Salt

Wet Ingredients

- 4 large Eggs

- 1 tsp Vanilla extract
- 1/2 tsp Stevia glycerite
- 2/3 cup Coconut milk (full fat)(158 ml)
- 3/4 large Granny Smith apple peeled, cored, and grated (5 oz/ 141 g)

Crumb Topping

- 1/3 cup of dry ingredients
- 1 tbsp of melted butter (ghee or coconut oil)
- 1 tbsp Granulated erythritol

Method

1. Preheat Oven to 325 °F. Line up the 12 cup muffin tin with the baking paper of the usual size.
2. Peel the Granny Smith apple.
3. Weigh 5 ounces and grate them (about 3/4 of a big apple).
4. In a medium cup, weigh all the dry ingredients and blend them to break up the lumps.
5. To use as the crumb topping, stir 1/3 cup of a mixture into a small dish.
6. Fill a large bowl with all the grated apple and wet ingredients.
7. Blend with the hand mixer.
8. Pour dry ingredients into wet ingredients and mix until they are combined.

Coconut Flour Chocolate Chip Cookies

Servings: 8

Time: 20 mins

Difficulty: Easy

Nutrients per serving: Calories: 71 kcal | Fat: 6.44g | Carbohydrates: 2.85g | Protein: 1.31g | Fiber: 2g

Ingredients

- 2 tbsp Low carb brown sugar (or your favorite granulated sweetener)
- 2 tbsp Light Olive Oil
- 2 tbsp Almond Butter or nut/seed butter of choice
- 1/4 cup Coconut Flour
- 1/2 tsp Vanilla Extract
- 1 tbsp Lily's Sugar-Free Chocolate Chips or 85-90% dark chocolate
- 1 tbsp Flax Meal
- 1 pinch Salt

Method

1. In a medium mixing cup, prepare the flax egg by stirring 1 tbsp of flax meal and 2.5 tbsp of water together. To thicken, leave for a few minutes.
2. Using a spatula, whisk in the vanilla extract and almond butter, and sunflower oil.
3. Add low-carb brown sugar, a touch of salt, and coconut flour to taste. To shape the dough, blend well.
4. Stir in the chips or bits of chocolate. Take 1 Tbsp. of cookie dough and roll your hands into a ball. Place the ball and flatten it into a cookie shape on a baking tray (the cookies will not spread - thinner cookies result in a crisper cookie).
5. Repeat for the cookie dough that remains.
6. At 350 F/ 180 C or until crispy around the outside, bake the cookies for about 15 minutes. Don't bake over them. Enjoy when fully refrigerated.
7. Store in the refrigerator in an airtight jar. Refrigerating mitigates the erythritol-based sweetener's cooling feeling.

Keto Chocolate Chia Pudding

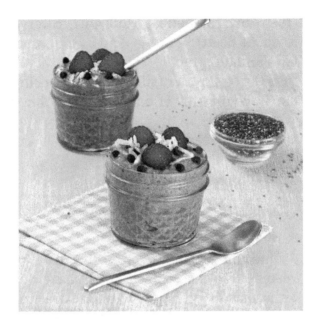

Servings: 2

Time: 35 mins

Difficulty: Easy

Nutrients per serving: Calories: 336 kcal | Fat: 27.3g | Carbohydrates: 16g | Protein: 8g | Fiber: 11g

Ingredients

- 2 tbsp low carb sugar (Sukrin:1, Swerve, Lakanto, Truvia, or Besti)
- 1 tsp Vanilla Extract
- 1 tbsp Cocoa Powder (sift before measuring)
- 1 cup Coconut Milk (from a can) (or Almond Milk for fewer calories)
- 1/4 cup Chia Seeds

Method

1. To a mason jar, apply the chocolate powder and sweetener. To clear some lumps, shake well.
2. To the mason jar, apply vanilla extract and coconut milk. tIn order to mix, close the lid, and then shake.
3. Apply to the jar the chia seeds and shake again. Move the container to the fridge until the mixture is well mixed.
4. For at least 30 min, cool it.
5. Serve a chocolate chia pudding with almond yogurt and seasonal fruit in your favorite jars.

Fluffy Keto Banana Cream Pie

Servings: 8

Time: 55 mins

Difficulty: Easy

Nutrients per serving: Calories: 526 kcal | Fat: 47g | Carbohydrates: 9.8g | Protein: 11g | Fiber: 4.3g

Ingredients

Low Carb Crust

- 1 recipe Low Carbohydrates Walnut Pie Crust

Banana Pudding (refrigerate overnight)

- 1 cup heavy cream
- 1 tbsp arrowroot powder
- 1 pinch salt
- 3 large egg yolks
- 2 large eggs
- 2 tbsp butter
- 1 tsp vanilla
- 1 tsp banana extract
- 1/2 cup low carb sugar (Swerve granulated or Lakanto)
- 1/3 cup almond milk

- 1 1/4 tsp gelatin powder
- 1/8 tsp xanthan gum

Whipped Cream (for folding into the Banana pudding)

- 2 tbsp low carb powdered sugar (or Swerve Confection or Lakanto Powdered)
- 1/8 tsp xanthan gum
- 1/2 cup heavy cream

Method

1. 1.Make the Low Carbohydrate Walnut Pie Crust according to the direction. Make it cool.
2. Ready by the stove for a strainer. To bloom, spray the gelatin over 1 Tbsp. of water.
3. In a medium saucepan, put the cream & almond milk, turn heat to medium before the milk steams, and create bubbles across the pan sides.
4. Whisk the arrowroot, sweetener, xanthan gum, and salt together in a medium dish. To mix, add the egg yolks or whole eggs and whisk.
5. Add the hot milk into the egg mixture in a thin stream while constantly whisking.

Low Carb Lemon Curd

Servings: 10

Time: 25 mins

Difficulty: Easy

Nutrients per serving: Calories: 120 kcal | Fat: 10.7g | Carbohydrates: 2.6g | Protein: 3.74g | Fiber: 0.1g

Ingredients

- 3/4 cup (6 ounces) lemon juice, about 3-4 large lemons
- 1/4 Tsp. stevia glycerite
- 1/2 cup low carb sugar (or Swerve, or Lakanto Monkfruit)
- 4 large eggs
- 4 large egg yolks
- the zest from all of the lemons
- 6 Tbsp. salted butter
- 1 Tbsp. arrowroot powder

Method

1. Weigh and put the erythritol and the arrowroot powder in a medium bath. Stir it together.
2. To make them juicy, roll the lemons on the table, then zest the lemons, applying the zest to erythritol.
3. Separate four eggs and apply the yolks to the pot of erythritol.
4. To the bowl, add the 4 whole eggs and whisk together the eggs and erythritol.
5. Juice and weigh 3/4 cup of the lemons.
6. Strain the juice from the lemon and whisk it into the eggs.
7. Down to medium-low, switch the heat, and finish whisking.

Low Carb Lemon Lush Dessert

Servings: 15

Time: 9 hrs 30 mins

Difficulty: Easy

Nutrients per serving: Calories: 308 kcal | Fat: 29g | Carbohydrates: 6.4g | Protein: 7g | Fiber: 1.9g

Ingredients

Lemon Curd (**Time:** 20 minutes)

1 recipe Lemon Curd (chilled at least 4 hours)

Shortbread Crust (**Time:** 30 minutes) (cool completely)

- 3/4 cup pecans, finely chopped
- 1/3 cup whey protein powder
- 1/3 cup of powdered sweetener (Swerve, Sukrin, or Lakanto)
- 2 cups almond flour
- 7 tbsp of salted butter (melted)

Cream Cheese Layers (**Time:** 10 minutes)

- 1 tsp vanilla extract
- 1/4 cup heavy whipping cream (2 fl oz)

- 1/4 cup powdered sweetener (Sukrin, Swerve, or Lakanto)
- 16 oz softened cream cheese (2 packages)

Heavy whipping cream (divided use) (**Time:** 10 minutes)

- 2 cups heavy whipping cream
- 2 tbsp powdered sweetener
- 1 tsp vanilla
- 1/8 tsp xanthan gum (optional - stabilizes the whipped cream)

Assembly (about 10 minutes)

Method

1. Before assembling the cake, prepare a lemon curd and allow it to cool fully for about 4 hours. It is possible to do this many days in advance. It is also excellent to make the shortbread crust ahead.

Pecan Shortbread Crust

1. Preheat the oven to 350 °F. Chop the pecans fairly fine and mix in a small bowl with the rest of the dry ingredients. To mix, whisk together. Melt the butter and pour the spices over it. To form a sticky, crumbly paste, combine with a fork.

2. Pour the materials into a pyrex baking dish of 13x9 inch glass and lay a waxed paper layer on the mixture. Use both fingertips, and press tightly into the bottom of a pan with

a flat bottom bottle or measurement cup. Remove a waxed paper, then bake for about 15 minutes, until softly golden.

Whipped Cream

Whip the vanilla and sweeteners with the milk until it is stiff.

Cream Cheese Layer

Whip the cream cheese until nice and light with 1/4 of heavy cream and a sweetener. Adding 1/2 cup of whipped cream at a time, fold 1 1/2 cups of the whipped cream into the cream cheese. Over a shortbread crust, spread evenly.

Lemon Curd Layer

1. When loosened, whisk the lemon curd and scatter softly over the cream cheese surface. Spread the leftover whipped cream gently over the lemon curd. It is better to refrigerate for several hours or overnight.

Sugar-Free Pecan Turtle Cheesecake Bars

Servings: 16

Time: 30 mins

Difficulty: Easy

Nutrients per serving: Calories: 439 kcal | Fat: 42g | Carbohydrates: 13g | Protein: 6g | Fiber: 8g

Ingredients

- 1 recipe Homemade Low Carbohydrates Caramel Sauce
- 1 recipe Low Carbohydrates Hot Fudge Sauce

Brown Sugar Pecan Crust
- 4 Tbsp. salted butter, (melted) (2 oz/ 57 g)
- 1/4 cup of whey protein powder (25 g)
- 1/3 cup of Sukrin Gold powdered (70 g)
- 1 cup toasted pecans, (ground) (4 oz/ 114 g)
- 1 cup of Almond Flour (4 oz / 114 g)

Vanilla Cheesecake
- 1 Tbsp. (15 g) vanilla extract

- 2 1/2 packages cream cheese, (softened) (20 oz / 567 g)
- 1/2 cup heavy cream, (whipped) (4 oz/ 118.29 ml)
- 1/2 Tsp. of Stevia Glycerite
- 2/3 cup of low carb powdered sugar (3 oz / 85 g)

<u>Topping</u>

- fudge sauce for drizzling
- caramel sauce for drizzling
- 1 cup toasted pecans, chopped (4 oz/ 114 g)

Method

1. Preheat the oven to 350 F and toast the pecans all.
2. Spray a 9X9 inch wide baking pan with baking spray and cover with a long enough parchment sheet such that two sides hang over it.
3. This will allow you to remove the bars for faster cutting and to serve in 1 big section.
4. 4.Grind the Sukrin Gold and add it to a medium bowl in a coffee grinder.
5. In a coffee grinder, grind the pecans and apply the sweetener to the medium dish.
6. Apply the remainder of the dry ingredients and thoroughly mix.
7. Melt and blend the butter into the dry ingredients.
8. When pressed softly in your palm, the mixture should stay together. In the microwave, heat the caramel and hot fudge sauces until soft and stir with a pour-able consistency.

Keto Sour Cream Cake

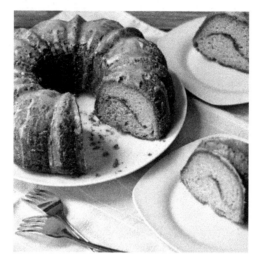

Servings: 12

Time: 50 mins

Difficulty: Easy

Nutrients per serving: Calories: 358 kcal | Fat: 34.5g | Carbohydrates: 7g | Protein: 8.6g | Fiber: 2.5g

Ingredients

Cake:

- 3 cups almond flour (280 g)

- 1 tsp sea salt
- 3 large eggs (I always use cold)
- 2 tsp vanilla extract
- 1/2 tsp baking soda
- 1/2 cup sour cream
- 1/2 tsp stevia glycerite
- 1/4 cup salted butter, melted (4 tbsp, 2 oz)
- 2/3 cup low carb sugar

Frosting:

- 6 oz cold cream cheese
- 3/4 cup heavy cream
- 1/4 tsp stevia glycerite
- 1/4 cup salted butter (very soft) (4 tbsp, 2 oz)
- 1/3 cup low carb powdered sugar
- 1 tsp vanilla extract

Garnish:

- 12 mint sprigs
- 36 small blueberries
- 6 medium strawberries, halved

Method

1. Preheat the oven to 350 F and place the rack in the center position. Spray a 1/4-sheet tray with baking spray (small jelly roll pan).
2. With parchment paper, line the bottom and spray a paper. Whisk the almond flour to break up some lumps before weighing with a whisk.

3. Measure into a medium-large bowl all the dry ingredients. Whisk to mix thoroughly. Add all the wet ingredients to dry ingredients and combine using a hand mixer thoroughly.
4. For the best results, spread the dense batter onto the ready sheet pan and smooth uniformly with an offset spatula.
5. Bake for 20-30 minutes. When gently pressed with a finger, the cake must spring back but still sound mildly moist. Remove from the oven and perfectly cool.
6. Place a cold cream cheese with the vanilla extract, powdered sweetener, and stevia glycerite in a small-medium cup.
7. Beat until the cream cheese is fully smooth and soft with a hand mixer, around 1-2 min, scraping down each side to remove any leftover lumps.

Keto Chocolate Mug Cake

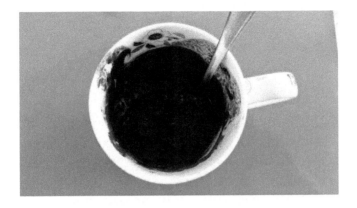

Servings: 1

Time: 3 mins

Difficulty: Easy

Nutrients per serving: Calories: 272 kcal | Fat: 23g | Carbohydrates: 7g | Protein: 9g | Fiber: 4g

Ingredients

- 1 large egg yolk
- 1 tbsp cocoa powder
- 1 tbsp low carb sugar (Lakanto or Swerve)
- 1 tbsp mayonnaise (use sour cream in a pinch)

- 1 tsp water
- 1/4 tsp baking powder
- 2 tbsp almond flour

Method

a. Until weighing, fluff up the almond flour with a whisk and sift before measuring the cocoa powder.
b. Measure into a mug or jelly jar the dry ingredients and blend fully with a fork.
c. Add the egg yolk, mayonnaise, and water, stirring thoroughly to make sure you have all from the bottom. Leave the batter to rest for 1-2 minutes.
d. Depending on the microwave, microwave for 50 seconds.

Lemon Ricotta Cake

Servings: 9

Time: 1 hr

Difficulty: Easy

Nutrients per serving: Calories: 212 kcal | Fat: 17g | Carbohydrates: 7g | Protein: 8g | Fiber: 3.5g

Ingredients

- 1/2 stick soft butter (2 oz/57 g)
- 1/2 cup low carb sugar (Swerve Granulated or Lakanto Classic)
- 1 1/2 tbsp fresh lemon juice
- 4 large eggs (cold) (one more egg if not using baking powder)
- 1 cup whole milk ricotta cheese (cold) (250 g)
- 1 tsp lemon zest (zest from one lemon)
- 1 tsp vanilla extract

Dry Ingredients
- 1 cup almond flour (whisk before measuring)
- 1/4 tsp salt
- 2 tsp baking powder

- 4 tbsp coconut flour (whisk before measuring)

Method

1. To 325 °F. Preheat oven. To suit the inner bottom of an 8 x 2-inch circular pan, cut a slice of parchment. The pan is sprayed or buttered, and the parchment is applied.
2. In a small dish, weigh the dry ingredients and whisk to remove any lumps—the cream when fully mixed with the butter, vanilla, and sweetener.
3. Add one egg and beat until fluffy and light. Stir in the ricotta cheese, lemon zest, lemon juice, and beat until well mixed.
4. Mix 1/3 of the dry ingredients into the batter by working by thirds.
5. Add the egg and blend. Repeat by starting with the last egg with the remaining ingredients. Carefully spread the batter with an offset spatula into the prepared cake tray.
6. Bake for 50 minutes or until the middle of the cake comes out clean with a toothpick inserted. Wrap every remaining cake in cling film and leave for 3 days (unless it is hot and humid) or refrigerate in the fridge.
7. Slightly warm before eating, if refrigerated.

Keto Strawberry Crepes

Servings: 4

Time: 15 mins

Difficulty: Easy

Nutrients per serving: Calories: 316 kcal | Fat: 29g | Carbohydrates: 5g | Protein: 9g | Fiber: 0.5g

Ingredients

- 4 low carb crepes
- 4 tbsp low carb sugar (divided use)
- 3 ounces fresh strawberries, quartered and sliced
- 2 tsp Brandy, Rum, or Bourbon (optional, replace with water)
- 2 tsp water
- 1/2 cup Heavy Whipping Cream
- 1/2 tsp vanilla extract
- 1/2 cup sour cream

Method

1. In a small bowl with 1 tbsp of the sweetener, apply the brandy and water, and combine to dissolve. It does not completely dissolve. Slice the strawberries, then put them in a small dish. Apply the combination of brandy and stir. Put the bowl aside as you macerate the strawberries.

2. In a 2-3 cup mug, weigh the heavy cream, the leftover sweetener, and vanilla. Whip until very rigid.

3. In a shallow dish, apply the sour cream and whisk it to loosen. Spoon 1/4 of whipped cream onto the sour cream and mix the cream softly. Fold half of the leftover whipped cream with a large spoon or rubber spatula onto the sour cream mixture. Apply to the sour cream mixture the leftover whipped cream and fold together fully. (At this point, the filling could be refrigerated for up to a day.) (Makes around 1 1/2 cups)

4. Place half of each crepe with 1/4 of a whipped cream mixture, spreading just half of each crepe. Fold the exposed half over the filled side, then fold, like a handkerchief, corner to corner. On each tray, position one. (If sealed and refrigerated, the crepes should be filled for many hours before serving.)

5. Whisk the strawberries over each loaded crepe and spoon 1/4 of strawberries and juice on them. Serve.

Hazelnut Creme Brulee

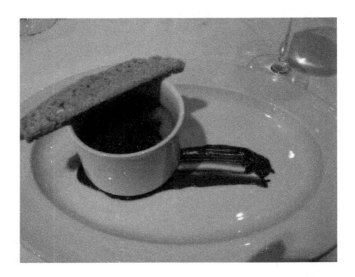

Servings: 2

Time: 40 mins

Difficulty: Easy

Nutrients per serving: Calories: 534 kcal | Fat: 52g | Carbohydrates: 4g | Protein: 7g

Ingredients

- 3 large egg yolks
- 2 tbsp spiced rum, brandy, or bourbon

- 2 tbsp low carb sugar (or Swerve Granular) (sugar, for non-low carbers)
- 1/4 tsp hazelnut extract
- 1 pinch salt
- 1 cup heavy cream

Optional (powdered sweetener for the top):
- 4 tsp Low carb brown sugar

Method

1. Preheat the oven to 350 °F and place the rack in the center position. Heat water until hot, not boiling, in a tea kettle. Halfway up the side of the ramekins, find a pan wide enough to accommodate 2, 6-oz ramekins and shallow enough to add water.
2. Add to a small bowl the yolks, and sweetener. With a fork, beat well to perfectly break up the yolks. Drop some giant chalazae.
3. In a small pot, pour the heavy cream and put it over medium heat. Stir with a whisk periodically before bubbles appear along the pot's edge, and the cream steams. Turn the heat off and start pouring the egg yolk into the mixture of the hot cream - very gently, in a thin stream, all the while whisking rapidly. Spiced rum (bourbon, brandy) and hazelnut extract are whisked in.
4. Divide the combination of creme brulee equally between the ramekins. Put the ramekins in the pan and fill the cooking pan with hot water halfway up the

ramekin's sides (not boiling). Place the pan carefully in the oven and bake for thirty min or until the creme brulee is only centered in the very middle. (Depending on the form of the ramekin.o, it may always be just a little bit wiggly in the middle

5. In the water bath, cool the hazelnut creme brulee for 30 minutes before transferring it to a rack to cool entirely. Cover and refrigerate for about 4 hours with plastic wrap, but it's best overnight.

6. Sprinkle 1 tsp sweetener or over the tops of each creme brulee before serving. Melt the sweetener until it caramelizes, turning brown with a culinary torch. Instead, add to the top a dollop of whipped cream. Serve.

Sugar-Free Chocolate Pie

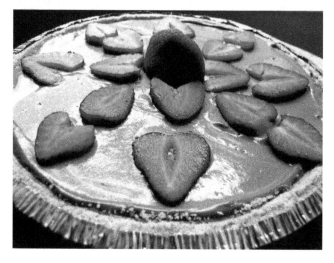

Servings: 10

Time: 40 mins

Difficulty: Easy

Nutrients per serving: Calories: 337 kcal | Fat: 34g | Carbohydrates: 8g | Protein: 6g | Fiber: 5g

Ingredients

Flaky Pie Crust

- 5 tbsp butter

- 3 tbsp oat fiber
- 1/4 tsp salt
- 1 tsp water
- 1 large egg white
- 1 1/2 cup almond flour

Filling

- 4 ounces unsweetened baking chocolate squares, melted
- 4 large pasteurized eggs, cold
- 2 Tsp. vanilla extract
- 6 ounces (1 1/2 sticks) salted butter, very soft
- 1/2 Tsp. stevia glycerite (or more Sukrin or Swerve to taste)
- 1 1/4 cups low carb powdered sugar (or Swerve Confectioners)
- 1/4 cup heavy cream

Topping

- chocolate shavings optional - I used 2 squares of Chocolate at 86% cacao
- 3/4 cup heavy cream
- 2 tbsp low carb powdered sugar (or swerve)

Method

1. Preheat the oven to 350°F. Using baking spray to spray a pie dish. I'm using a pyrex 9-inch baking dish. (On the pie plate base, we scatter sesame seeds, so the crust should not adhere to the bottom.)

2. Measure into the food processor the oat fiber, almond flour, and salt. Cut the butter into pellets and pulse with dry ingredients until the small peas are the butter's size. Mix 1 Tsp. of water with the white egg and spill over the dry ingredients. The phase before it all comes along with the dough. For about 30 minutes to 5 days, you can refrigerate the dough.
3. For your pie plate, roll the pastry into two sheets of plastic wrap until it becomes the right size. Remove the plastic top piece and invert dough over the plate of the pie. Coax the dough softly onto the bottom and sides of a plate. Remove the plastic and bring the edge into shape. With a fork, dock the dough.
4. Bake the crust for 10-15 minutes before the golden brown starts to transform. Let it cool fully, then cover until ready to use with plastic wrap.
5. Unsweetened baking chocolate is finely diced and stored in a microwaveable dish. Heat up to 30 secs at a time before it nearly melts. The excess heat from a bowl should ensure that the remainder is dissolved.
6. In a stand mixer or a large mixing cup, place the butter and Swerve or Sukrin Melis. Apply the paddle attachment to the mixer, then beat the butter and a sweetener for around 2 minutes at medium speed. Give the bowl a scrape. Add the chocolate to the molten one and blend for 1 minute. Scrape thoroughly down the bowl. Apply 1/4 cup of heavy cream, vanilla, then glycerin stevia, and beat for 2 more minutes. Spread a filling back into a bowl and drop the paddle attachment.
7. Add the whisk attachment and switch back at medium speed on the stand mixer. Add one egg on time and let the mixer run between each addition for about 3

minutes, scraping the pan after the third and fourth additions.

8. Finish blending at high speed with a fast burst and disperse the filling into the pie's shell and refrigerate. [NOTE: refrigerate for 40 minutes if the filling splits (separates), then add 1/4 tsp of xanthan gum. Whip to release the filling for a few seconds at medium speed and then at high just a few seconds before it comes together. There could be another pinch of xanthan gum if required.]

9. With a spoon or spatula, spoon the filling onto the pie crust, then smooth it. Refrigerate, and leave open for 6 hours or overnight.

10. Whip the 3/4 cup heavy cream and finish the pie with your preferred sweetener. Additionally, by running the vegetable peeler down of a chocolate slice, chocolate curls may be added.

Sugar-free Nutella Swirl Muffins

Servings: 6

Time: 40 mins

Difficulty: Easy

Nutrients per serving: Calories: 255 kcal | Fat: 22g | Carbohydrates: 6g | Protein: 9g | Fiber: 1g

Ingredients

<u>Dry Ingredients</u>

- 1/4 tsp salt
- 1 tsp baking powder
- 1 tbsp whey protein powder (We use Isopure Zero Carb)
- 1 1/2 cups Almond Flour (130 g)

<u>Wet Ingredients</u>

- 2 large eggs
- 1/2 cup heavy cream
- 1 1/2 tsp vanilla extract
- 1/3 cup low carb sugar

<u>Swirl Topping</u>

- 6 tsp Free Chocolate Hazelnut Spread (Sukrin Sugar)

Method

1. Preheat the oven to 350 F and put the rack in the center position. Strip 6 muffin wells of standard size with parchment liners. In the microwave, heat a Sukrin Chocolate Hazelnut Spread for 20-30 seconds or until a Tsp. is easy to drizzle.
2. Place the wet ingredients in the mixer. Place the dry ingredients in the mixer then. Switch down the mixer and mix. With a spatula, cut the lid and help the phase-out. Turn to medium-low and mix for 20 seconds just until the batter is smooth and well ventilated.
3. Divide the muffin batter, filling 3/4 full, among six muffin wells. Drizzle 1 Tsp. of Sukrin Chocolate Hazelnut Spread and swirl/mix with a toothpick over each muffin.
4. Bake for about 25-35 minutes or until the muffin tops are smooth to the touch and springy but still sound moist. Cool in the muffin tin for 5 minutes, then remove from a cooling rack. Refrigerate for 7-10 days in an airtight jar or stock for up to 5 days on the fridge.

Moist Chocolate Walnut Cake

Servings: 12

Time: 55 mins

Difficulty: Easy

Nutrients per serving: Calories: 264 kcal | Fat: 23g | Carbohydrates: 10g | Protein: 8g | Fiber: 5g

Ingredients

<u>Dry Ingredients</u>

- 3 ounces walnuts
- 1/4 Tsp. salt
- 1/3 cup coconut flour (fluff up with whisk before measuring)
- 1/3 cup cocoa powder (sift then measure)
- 1/2 cup low carb sugar (or Swerve Granulated)
- 1 tbsp baking powder
- 1 1/4 cup almond flour (whisk before measuring)

<u>Wet Ingredients</u>

- 4 large eggs
- 1 Tsp. vanilla
- 1 Tsp. stevia glycerite

- 1/2 cup buttermilk (or heavy cream or full-fat coconut milk)
- 1/4 cup walnut oil (or melted butter)

Chocolate Ganache Glaze

- 1/4 cup heavy cream
- 2 oz Ghiradelli Intense Dark Chocolate (86% or any high percentage chocolate)
- 2 Tbsp. butter or coconut oil (room temperature)

Method

a. Preheat the oven to 325 ℉ and put the rack in the center of the oven. On the sheet of waxed paper or the parchment, trace the base of an 8 x 2 inches cake tray. Cut the circle out. Spray the cake pan with the baking spray and line the parchment circle at the pan's bottom. Weigh the walnuts and grind the sweetener until finely ground in a food processor.

b. In a medium cup, weigh the dry cake ingredients (along with ground walnuts) and vigorously stir with a large whisk to mix. Add the wet ingredients to another bowl and pound them with a hand mixer. Add the wet ingredients to the dry dish and combine until all the ingredients are thoroughly integrated.

c. To dislodge some large air bubbles, spoon the batter in the cake pan and softly tap it on a counter 2-3 times. When carefully squeezed with your finger and insert a toothpick in the middle, bake for about 30-40 minutes or until the cake still looks moist. Do not bake in excess.

d. Take a Chocolate Walnut Cake from the oven and cover it with a clean tea towel. Let the cake perfectly cold. Then seal until ready to cover with ganache in plastic wrap. Until topping with the ganache, ensure that the cake is at room temperature.

e. Finely cut the chocolate and put it with the heavy cream and butter in a shallow microwaveable dish. Cover with waxed paper, then microwave for 30 seconds. For 1 minute, let stand, then gently whisk to mix. The ganache should be rich and shiny. Use it instantly.

f. Pour a chocolate ganache in the middle of a cake and spread it over the side with a spatula or knife, causing it to spill. Decorate, if you wish, with walnut halves (optional) or pieces of walnut while the ganache is still moist. Once the ganache has set, cut, and serve (it will still be fairly soft but not runny).

g. Hold it in the fridge or on the table. Let it arrive at room temperature for about 30 minutes before having it if refrigerated.

Blackberry Custard Pie

Servings: 10

Time: 20 mins

Difficulty: Easy

Nutrients per serving: Calories: 357 kcal | Fat: 32g | Carbohydrates: 8g | Protein: 11g | Fiber: 3g

Ingredients

- 4 large eggs
- 3/4 cup heavy cream
- 2 large egg yolks
- 1/4 tsp xanthan gum
- 1/2 cup low carb sugar
- 1 tsp vanilla extract
- 1 tsp gelatin powder (flourished in 1 tbsp water)
- 1 recipe Low Carbohydrates Keto Graham Cracker Crust (resists soaking)
- 1 pinch salt
- 1 pinch ground nutmeg
- 1 cup buttermilk
- 1 cup blackberries (1/2 pint)

Method

1. To bloom, sprinkle gelatin with 1 Tbsp. of water. Measure the sweetener, xanthan gum, and salt in a non-reactive metal pot with a 4-6 cup size. Add the yolks and eggs and mix until thoroughly mixed. Whisk in the heavy cream and buttermilk.

2. Put the pot over medium heat until the mixture starts to thicken, whisking continuously - about 5 minutes if using Tagatesse (either a sugar) and 8 mins for Sukrin:1 or Swerve. Switch the heat medium-low and whisk for 1 minute with vigor (If whisking fails, the custard can burst). Remove from the heat and whisk for 90 seconds more. Tear the gelatin into bits and pour it into the custard and stir until it is dissolved. Include vanilla and the nutmeg, stirring until combined.

3. Only cool the mixture slowly, and pipe it onto the pre-baked pie crust. Balance the top and layer the blackberries until they are at least halfway submerged, pressing them into a custard. Refrigerate exposed before coating with cling film for several hours. Before chopping and serving, chill for at least 6 hours.

Low Carb Chocolate Chip Muffins

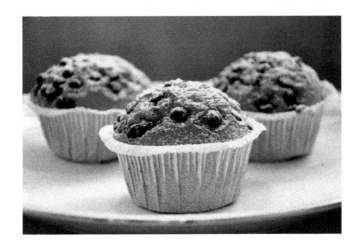

Servings: 6

Time: 30 mins

Difficulty: Easy

Nutrients per serving: Calories: 270 kcal | Fat: 24g | Carbohydrates: 11g | Protein: 7g | Fiber: 7g

Ingredients

Cream Together:
- 1/2 tsp of lemon zest
- 1/2 tsp of vanilla extract

- 1/4 cup low carb sugar
- 2 oz softened unsalted butter
- 4 oz softened cream cheese

Dry Ingredients:

- 1 tsp baking powder
- 1/2 cup coconut flour
- 1/4 tsp salt
- 1/8 tsp xanthan gum

Wet Ingredients:

- 1/4 cup heavy cream
- 3 large eggs

Fold:

- 3 tbsp Lily's Sugar-free Chocolate Chips
- 4 oz strawberries, small dice

Method

1. Preheat the oven to 350 °F and place the rack in the middle. Standard muffin wells from Line 6 with paper liners. Dice some strawberries. The lemon zest. Mix the dry ingredients.
2. Cream together the whole 5 ingredients until light and smooth with a hand mixer. Again, add 1 egg and milk.
3. Apply 1/3 of the dry, well-beaten ingredients, followed by another egg. Only repeat. Make sure that a soft

mousse-like appearance is preserved by fading out. The rest of the dry ingredients are added, followed by heavy cream. Half of the strawberries and half of the chocolate chips are rolled in. The batter's going to be dense.

4. Spoon the batter in a zip-lock bag and slit one of the corners with a wide hole. Squeeze the batter, placed in the middle, onto each liner. Use a muffin scoop alternately. To resist browning, brush the top of the muffins with erythritol. Arrange the remaining chocolate chips and strawberries on top.

5. In the oven center, put the muffin tin and set the oven up to 400 °F for 6 minutes. Switch the oven back to 350 °F and bake for an extra 12-18 minutes. The tops should be solid to the touch but still, look a little wet. On a wire rack, cool perfectly. Keep it softly warm in the refrigerator before eating it.

No-Bake Sugar-Free Strawberry Cheesecake Tart

Servings: 10

Time: 35 mins

Difficulty: Easy

Nutrients per serving: Calories: 306 kcal | Fat: 28g | Carbohydrates: 5g | Protein: 10g | Fiber: 3g

Ingredients

Walnut Hemp Seeds Crust
- 2 tbsp of coconut oil (melted)
- 1/2 cup Bob's Mill Hemp Seed's Hearts
- 1 tbsp of Sukrin Fiber Gold Syrup/Vitafiber Syrup
- 1 cup walnut pieces, toasted

Cheesecake Filling
- 1 tbsp lemon juice
- 1/4 cup low carb powdered sugar
- 4 ounces cream cheese cold
- 4 ounces softened goat cheese
- 6 ounces strawberries, sliced
- zest from the lemon

- 4 ounces heavy cream, cold

Optional

- 2 tsp fresh thyme or rosemary (finely chopped)

Method

1. The oven should be preheated to 350 °F. Put on a sheet pan and then toast the walnuts for 15 minutes or until golden in color. To remove most of the loosened skin, let it cool, then rub in the tea towel.

2. In a food processor, position the hemp seeds and the walnuts and grind them until finely ground. To spread the ingredients, apply the molten coconut oil and fiber syrup (you can use honey if not low carb), then pulse. (If rolled into balls, this also produces a perfect snack.)

3. Using parchment paper to cover a tart pan. (I used a round 14x6x1 tin, but it would fit with a big circular or many small round tins.) Spread the mixture of the crust into the pan and then force it into the crust to ensure that the sides are solid. Cover tightly and place until set in the freezer and the filling is prepared or place until appropriate in the refrigerator. It thaws rapidly.

4. In a cup, add cream cheese and the sweetener, and whip until loosened with a hand mixture. Add some heavy cream, then whip until soft and light. Finally, add the cheese from the goat and whip it again. Use or cover immediately and put in the fridge until needed. Whip to loosen before expanding onto the tart crust

when kept overnight in the refrigerator. (Place 1/3 of a filling in a piping bag before piping to decorate the roof. First, we place the strawberries and decorate them around.)

5. Cut the strawberries and add the filling to them. Serve instantly. If you serve later, right before eating, apply the sliced strawberries to keep them from being soggy.

Lightning Source UK Ltd.
Milton Keynes UK
UKHW021306060521
383235UK00005B/101